The Expectant Dad's Handbook

Navigating the Journey to Fatherhood

By

Eleanor Alva

TABLE OF CONTENTS

INTRODUCTION

We're glad you're here to learn about "The Expectant Dad's Handbook: Navigating the Journey to Fatherhood." I am honored to give this complete manual created especially for expectant fathers like you as a parenting and fatherhood expert. Congratulations on starting the life-changing and extraordinary path of fatherhood!

The experience of becoming a parent is amazing and transformative, and the expectant father's contribution is essential to laying a solid foundation for the future of the family. This book is written to equip you with the fundamental information, useful suggestions, and insightful knowledge you need to confidently and gracefully navigate the many stages of pregnancy, childbirth, and early motherhood.

We will examine the special difficulties and rewards that come with being a father-to-be in this handbook. From the exhilarating moment of discovering the pregnancy to preparing for the baby's arrival, we will explore every aspect of this transformative process together.

My objective as an expert is to be your go-to guide as we navigate the highs and lows, successes and failures of fatherhood. Each chapter is designed to cover a particular topic of interest, from understanding pregnancy and helping your partner to creating a successful parenting team and embracing fatherhood.

You will learn how to foster a loving atmosphere for your spouse and your unborn kid, how to participate actively in the labor and delivery process, and how to form a strong emotional connection with your unborn child. Additionally, as you embrace this new chapter in your life, we will discuss the significance of self-care, work-life balance, and cultivating your emotional wellbeing.

I want to urge you to be open, curious, and kind to yourself and your spouse along this journey. Accept the difficulties, rejoice in the victories, and never forget that fatherhood is a lifelong process of development.

More than just a book, The Expectant Dad's Handbook is a sincere and skillfully designed resource that will provide you the information and encouragement you need to embrace fatherhood with love, dedication, and assurance. Know that you are not alone, and that this guide is here to walk with you every step of the way, whether you are feeling anticipation, excitement, or even brief moments of anxiety.

I'm thrilled to be a part of your journey as a fatherhood expert, and I hope that this book proves to be a priceless source of inspiration and direction as you travel the lovely and transformational road to parenthood. May it serve as a guiding light and source of encouragement as you embrace the joys, difficulties, and wonders of fatherhood. Let's start out on this amazing journey together!

CHAPTER 1

THE EXCITEMENT BEGINS – (*Embracing The Journey To Fatherhood*)

The moment you discover that you are going to be a father is a blend of excitement, joy, and anticipation like no other. This chapter explores the beginning of your journey as an expectant father, from the exhilarating news to the emotions that fill your heart. It's a time of preparation, bonding, and envisioning the future with your growing family. Embrace the emotions that arise as you embark on this beautiful adventure, for the excitement of fatherhood is just the beginning of a remarkable and transformative experience.

1. The Joyful Revelation: Embracing the News

The moment your partner shares the news that you are going to be a father, an overwhelming wave of joy and excitement washes over you. The realization that you will soon hold a tiny life in your arms is both exhilarating and humbling. Embrace the joy and celebrate this milestone with your partner, knowing that your lives are about to change in the most beautiful way.

2. Anticipation and Preparation: Getting Ready for Fatherhood

As the reality of impending fatherhood settles in, anticipation and preparation become your companions. From setting up the nursery to reading parenting books, each step is an act of love and dedication to your growing family. Embrace the journey of preparing for fatherhood, knowing that every effort brings you closer to the moment you will hold your child in your arms.

3. Bonding with Your Partner: Navigating Parenthood Together

Expectant fatherhood is not just about you; it's a shared journey with your partner. Embrace the opportunity to deepen your bond as you navigate parenthood together. Attend prenatal classes, accompany your partner to doctor's appointments, and engage in heartfelt conversations about your hopes and dreams for your child. Building a strong foundation of support and understanding prepares you for the adventure ahead.

4. *Embracing the Emotions: From Excitement to Apprehension*

As an expectant father, a myriad of emotions floods your heart. From excitement and anticipation to moments of apprehension and uncertainty, know that it is normal to experience a range of feelings. Embrace these emotions, allowing yourself to process and understand them. Sharing your feelings with your partner or seeking support from other expectant fathers can provide valuable reassurance during this transformative time.

5. *Envisioning the Future: Dreams of Fatherhood*

As you embark on this journey, allow yourself to dream and envision the future with your child. Picture the moments you will share, the laughter and love that will fill your home, and the memories you will create together. Embracing these dreams ignites a profound sense of purpose and excitement, guiding you as you take each step toward fatherhood.

The excitement of expectant fatherhood marks the beginning of a remarkable and transformative journey. Embrace the joy, anticipation, and emotions that fill your heart as you prepare to welcome your child into the world. This chapter is a testament to the love and dedication you already possess, and it sets the stage for the adventure of a lifetime.

As you embark on this path, remember that each step is a celebration of love and family. Embrace the excitement that surrounds you, for fatherhood is a journey that will forever enrich your life and the lives of those you hold dear. Embrace the excitement, for it is just the beginning of a remarkable and transformative experience.

CHAPTER 2

UNDERSTANDING PREGNANCY -
Navigating the Journey with Knowledge and Support

Understanding pregnancy is an essential aspect of expectant fatherhood. This chapter explores the transformative journey of pregnancy, from conception to childbirth, as you navigate this new territory with knowledge and support. As an expectant father, being informed about the physical and emotional changes your partner experiences empowers you to be a steadfast and supportive presence during this significant time. Embrace the journey of understanding pregnancy, for it is a shared experience that deepens your bond and lays the foundation for the arrival of your precious child.

1. Conception and Early Pregnancy: The Miracle of Life Begins

The journey of pregnancy begins with conception, the miraculous moment when an egg and sperm unite to form a new life. As an expectant father, learning about the early stages of pregnancy allows you to witness the development of your child from the very beginning. Embrace the awe and wonder of this process, as you both create the foundation for a new life together.

2. The Physical Changes: Supporting Your Partner's Health

Pregnancy brings significant physical changes to your partner's body. From morning sickness and fatigue to hormonal fluctuations, understanding these changes allows you to be a caring and empathetic source of support. Attend prenatal appointments, offer healthy meals, and be attentive to your partner's needs as she navigates the physical aspects of pregnancy.

3. Emotional Support: Nurturing Your Partner's Well-Being

Pregnancy can also bring about emotional shifts and heightened sensitivity. As an expectant father, being emotionally attuned to your partner's feelings and providing a nurturing presence is paramount. Create an environment where she feels safe to express her emotions and share her thoughts, knowing that your support strengthens your bond as you navigate this journey together.

4. The Prenatal Experience: Attending Classes and Workshops

Embrace the opportunity to attend prenatal classes and workshops with your partner. These educational sessions provide valuable insights into pregnancy, childbirth, and newborn care. Participating together strengthens your partnership as you both prepare for the arrival of your child.

5. Preparing for Birth: Discussing Birth Plans and Preferences

Discussing birth plans and preferences with your partner is essential to ensure that her wishes are respected during labor and delivery. Understanding the options available and being actively involved in these discussions empowers you to be a supportive advocate during the birthing process.

6. A Shared Journey: Celebrating Milestones and Creating Memories

Throughout pregnancy, celebrate milestones and create cherished memories together. From hearing the baby's heartbeat for the first time to feeling the baby's kicks, each moment is a beautiful reminder of the life growing within. Embrace the shared journey, knowing that these experiences strengthen the connection with your partner and your growing child.

Understanding pregnancy is a fundamental aspect of expectant fatherhood. Embrace the journey with knowledge and support, as it deepens your bond with your partner and prepares you for the arrival of your child.

Being informed about the physical and emotional changes your partner experiences allows you to be a compassionate and attentive source of support. Participating in prenatal classes and discussions about birth plans empowers you to be an active advocate during the labor and delivery process.

Celebrate milestones and create cherished memories together, for pregnancy is a shared journey that shapes the foundation of your growing family. As you understand and embrace this transformative time, your love and support become the bedrock of a beautiful and connected parenting journey that lies ahead.

CHAPTER 3

SUPPORTING YOUR PARTNER -
Nurturing with Love and Understanding

Supporting your partner during pregnancy is a vital role as an expectant father. This chapter explores the significance of being a nurturing and understanding presence as your partner experiences the physical and emotional changes of pregnancy. From providing practical assistance to offering emotional support, your involvement is instrumental in creating a safe and loving environment for both your partner and the growing baby. Embrace the opportunity to be an unwavering pillar of support, for your care and love will make this journey all the more beautiful and memorable.

1. Attend Prenatal Appointments Together: Sharing the Journey

Accompanying your partner to prenatal appointments is a meaningful way to be actively involved in the pregnancy journey. These visits provide crucial insights into the baby's development and health. Your presence at appointments demonstrates your commitment to being a supportive and attentive partner.

2. Offer Physical Assistance: Lightening the Load

As pregnancy progresses, your partner may experience physical discomfort and fatigue. Offering a helping hand with household chores, cooking, or running errands lightens her load and allows her to focus on self-care and the well-being of the baby.

3. Be Empathetic and Understanding: Emotional Support Matters

Pregnancy can bring about a range of emotions, from joy and excitement to moments of anxiety and uncertainty. Be empathetic and understanding, providing a safe space for your partner to express her feelings. Listening attentively and offering reassurance strengthens the emotional bond between you both.

4. Educate Yourself: Understanding Pregnancy and Labor

Take the time to educate yourself about the various stages of pregnancy and labor. Being informed empowers you to actively participate in discussions with healthcare providers and support your partner in making informed decisions about her pregnancy and childbirth preferences.

5. Create Moments of Relaxation: Pampering and Caring

Treat your partner to moments of relaxation and pampering. A soothing massage, a warm bath, or a peaceful walk in nature can help alleviate stress and promote a sense of well-being. These gestures of care demonstrate your love and consideration.

6. Be Patient and Flexible: Adapt to Changing Needs

Pregnancy is a transformative journey, and your partner's needs may change as the months progress. Be patient and flexible, adapting to her evolving requirements. Your willingness to accommodate her changing needs shows your dedication and commitment as a partner.

7. *Celebrate Milestones: Cherishing the Journey*

Celebrate the milestones of pregnancy together. From the first ultrasound image to feeling the baby's movements, each moment is a celebration of life and love. Marking these occasions with joy and gratitude strengthens your bond as expectant parents.

<u>NOTE</u>:

Supporting your partner during pregnancy is a profound expression of love and commitment. Being actively involved in prenatal appointments, offering physical assistance, and providing emotional support create a nurturing and loving environment for your partner and the growing baby.

Educating yourself about pregnancy and labor empowers you to be an informed and involved partner. Creating moments of relaxation and celebration allows you both to cherish this transformative journey together.

Embrace the role of a supportive and understanding partner, for your love and care make all the difference in creating a beautiful and memorable pregnancy experience. Your dedication lays the foundation for a loving and connected parenting journey that extends well beyond pregnancy.

CHAPTER 4

PREPARING FOR PARENTHOOD -
Building a Strong Foundation for Your Family's Future

Preparing for parenthood is a transformative phase that lays the groundwork for a loving and nurturing family. This chapter explores the various aspects of getting ready to welcome your child into the world. From creating a supportive environment to learning essential parenting skills, the journey of preparation strengthens your bond as a couple and fosters a sense of readiness for the responsibilities of parenthood. Embrace the process of preparing for this new chapter in your life, knowing that the foundation you build will shape the trajectory of your family's future.

1. Communicating as Partners: Sharing Dreams and Concerns

Open and honest communication as partners is crucial when preparing for parenthood. Take the time to share your dreams, concerns, and expectations about parenting. Discuss your parenting philosophies and how you both envision raising your child. These conversations lay the groundwork for a unified approach to parenthood.

2. Attending Parenting Classes: Learning Together

Attending parenting classes is a valuable way to gain knowledge and skills as expectant parents. These classes cover essential topics such as newborn care, infant CPR, and breastfeeding. Learning together as a couple enhances your confidence and preparedness for the arrival of your child.

3. Establishing a Support System: Seeking Guidance and Assistance

Building a support system is essential as you prepare for parenthood. Seek guidance and advice from experienced parents, friends, or family members. Having a network of support provides reassurance and practical assistance during the early stages of parenting.

4. Preparing the Home: Creating a Safe and Nurturing Space

Transforming your home into a safe and nurturing space for your child is an essential aspect of preparation. Baby-proofing the house, setting up the nursery, and organizing baby essentials are significant steps in ensuring your home is ready for the new arrival.

5. Budgeting and Financial Planning: Preparing for New Responsibilities

Parenthood brings new financial responsibilities. Take the time to review your budget and financial plan, considering expenses related to medical care, baby supplies, and childcare. Planning ahead ensures a stable foundation for your family's financial well-being.

6. Exploring Parental Leave and Work-Life Balance: Prioritizing Family

Discuss parental leave and work-life balance with your employer to create a plan that allows both parents to be present during the early stages of parenthood. Balancing work and family life is essential for fostering a supportive and nurturing environment for your child.

7. *Embracing the Journey: Anticipating the Joys and Challenges*

Preparing for parenthood is an adventure filled with anticipation and excitement. Embrace the journey, knowing that it will be filled with moments of joy, growth, and challenges. Your willingness to embrace the unknown and work together as a team sets the stage for a positive and rewarding parenting experience.

<u>NOTE:</u>

Preparing for parenthood is a transformative phase that strengthens your bond as a couple and builds a strong foundation for your family's future. Communicating openly, attending parenting classes, and establishing a support system are essential steps in preparing for the responsibilities of parenthood.

Creating a safe and nurturing home, planning financially, and prioritizing work-life balance contribute to a stable and supportive environment for your child. Embrace the journey with anticipation and excitement, knowing that the love and dedication you invest in preparing for parenthood will shape the beautiful and meaningful experience that lies ahead.

CHAPTER 5

HEALTH AND WELLNESS -
Nurturing a Healthy Start for Your Child

Health and wellness are paramount considerations as you prepare to welcome your child into the world. This chapter delves into the essential aspects of maintaining the physical and emotional well-being of both expectant parents and the growing baby. From prenatal care and nutrition to managing stress and promoting mental well-being, nurturing a healthy start sets the foundation for a thriving and vibrant family. Embrace the journey of prioritizing health and wellness, knowing that it contributes to a positive and nurturing environment for your child's development.

1. Prenatal Care: Navigating the Journey with Professional Support

Prenatal care is an integral part of a healthy pregnancy. Regular visits to healthcare providers ensure that both your partner's and the baby's health are closely monitored. Embrace these visits as an opportunity to gain insights into the baby's development and address any concerns you may have as expectant parents.

2. Nutrition and Healthy Eating: Fueling Growth and Development

Maintaining a balanced and nutritious diet is essential during pregnancy. Ensure that your partner is consuming a variety of fruits, vegetables, lean proteins, and whole grains. Proper nutrition provides essential nutrients for the baby's growth and supports your partner's well-being.

3. Physical Activity: Embracing Safe Exercise

Regular physical activity benefits both expectant parents and the baby. Encourage your partner to engage in safe exercises approved by healthcare professionals, such as prenatal yoga or swimming. Physical activity helps reduce stress, improves sleep, and promotes a healthy pregnancy.

4. Managing Stress: Fostering Emotional Well-Being

Pregnancy can bring about moments of stress and anxiety. Encourage open communication with your partner, creating a safe space for her to share her feelings. Engaging in relaxation techniques, such as deep breathing or meditation, can also help manage stress during this transformative time.

5. Sleep and Rest: Prioritizing Restorative Sleep

Adequate sleep and rest are essential for expectant parents' well-being. Encourage a regular sleep schedule and create a relaxing sleep environment to promote restorative rest. Support your partner in finding comfortable sleeping positions that accommodate her growing belly.

6. Mental Health: Recognizing the Importance of Emotional Support

Mental health is a significant aspect of overall wellness. Be attentive to your partner's emotional well-being, offering reassurance and understanding. Seek professional support if needed, ensuring that she has access to the resources to maintain good mental health throughout pregnancy.

7. Bonding with Your Baby: Connecting in the Womb

Encourage bonding with your baby by talking, reading, and singing to the growing bump. Engaging in these activities fosters a sense of connection and familiarity for both expectant parents and the baby.

Conclusion:

Health and wellness are foundational elements as you prepare to welcome your child into the world. Prioritizing prenatal care, nutrition, and physical activity creates a healthy environment for the baby's growth and development.

Managing stress, promoting emotional well-being, and nurturing mental health support your partner's overall wellness. Bonding with your baby in the womb fosters a strong connection that extends beyond birth.

Embrace the journey of nurturing health and wellness, knowing that the love and care you invest in these essential aspects contribute to a thriving and vibrant family dynamic. The journey of nurturing health and wellness sets the foundation for a positive and nurturing environment for your child's development. Embrace the journey of prioritizing health and wellness, for it is a testament to the love and care you have for your growing family.

CHAPTER 6

BONDING WITH YOUR UNBORN CHILD - Embracing the Miracle of Connection

Bonding with your unborn child is a precious and transformative experience for expectant fathers. This chapter delves into the various ways you can establish a deep and meaningful connection with your baby before they even arrive. From talking and singing to your growing belly to actively participating in prenatal activities, bonding with your unborn child lays the foundation for a strong and loving parent-child relationship. Embrace the journey of nurturing this unique connection, knowing that your love and presence create a profound impact on your child's early development.

1. Talking and Singing to Your Baby: The Power of Your Voice

Your voice is a comforting and familiar sound to your unborn child. Engage in conversations and sing gentle lullabies, allowing your baby to recognize your voice even before birth. This practice fosters a sense of security and connection between you and your child.

2. Feeling the Baby's Movements: Shared Moments of Joy

As your partner experiences the baby's movements, actively participate in feeling the kicks and hiccups. These shared moments of joy strengthen the bond between you, your partner, and your growing baby. Place your hand on the belly and marvel at the miracle of life.

3. Attending Prenatal Appointments Together: Shared Involvement

Accompanying your partner to prenatal appointments provides valuable opportunities for bonding with your unborn child. Listening to the baby's heartbeat or seeing ultrasound images creates an emotional connection that extends beyond words.

4. Reading Stories and Playing Music: Nurturing Early Stimulation

Reading stories or playing soft music to your baby in the womb fosters early stimulation and cognitive development. Your voice and choice of music create a soothing environment that nurtures your baby's senses.

5. *Creating a Welcoming Nursery: Preparing for Their Arrival*

As you prepare the nursery, involve yourself in the process of creating a welcoming and nurturing space for your child. As you assemble the crib and decorate the room, your anticipation and excitement become tangible expressions of your love.

6. *Writing Letters or Keeping a Journal: Expressing Your Emotions*

Writing letters or keeping a journal addressed to your unborn child is a beautiful way to express your emotions and hopes for their future. This practice allows you to articulate your love and dedication, creating a cherished keepsake for your child to treasure in the years to come.

7. *Bonding with Your Partner: Embracing Parenthood Together*

Bonding with your unborn child is also about deepening your connection with your partner. Engage in conversations about your feelings, hopes, and dreams as you both anticipate the arrival of your baby. Supporting each other during this transformative time strengthens your partnership and the love you will share as parents.

Conclusion:

Bonding with your unborn child is a profound and heartwarming experience for expectant fathers. Talking and singing to your baby, feeling their movements, and attending prenatal appointments together all contribute to nurturing this unique connection.

Reading stories, playing music, and creating a welcoming nursery prepares your baby for their arrival into a loving home. Writing letters or keeping a journal is a touching way to express your emotions and dedication.

Embrace the journey of bonding with your unborn child, for it is a beautiful foundation for the strong and loving parent-child relationship that will flourish in the years to come. Your love, presence, and anticipation create a profound impact on your child's early development, fostering a sense of security and connection that will last a lifetime.

CHAPTER 7

PREPARING FOR LABOR AND DELIVERY - Supporting Your Partner through the Birthing Journey

Preparing for labor and delivery is an essential aspect of expectant fatherhood. This chapter delves into the various ways you can support your partner during this transformative and momentous event. From attending childbirth education classes to creating a birthing plan, your involvement and encouragement play a crucial role in helping your partner feel empowered and prepared for the birthing process. Embrace the journey of preparing for labor and delivery, knowing that your presence and support create a positive and nurturing environment for both your partner and your baby.

1. Childbirth Education: Gaining Knowledge Together

Attending childbirth education classes as a couple is a valuable way to gain knowledge and insights into the birthing process. Understanding the stages of labor, pain management options, and the role of a supportive partner empowers you to actively participate and assist during the delivery.

2. Creating a Birth Plan: Discussing Preferences and Choices

Working with your partner to create a birth plan allows both of you to express your preferences and choices for the labor and delivery experience. Discuss pain relief options, medical interventions, and any specific desires your partner may have for the birthing process.

3. Practicing Breathing Techniques: Calming and Comforting

Breathing techniques are a useful tool to help your partner stay calm and relaxed during labor. Practice deep breathing exercises together to familiarize yourselves with the techniques and use them as a means of support during the birthing process.

4. Assembling a Birthing Bag: Being Prepared for the Big Day

Prepare a birthing bag with essential items for both your partner and yourself. Include comfortable clothing, snacks, water bottles, and any comforting items that may help during labor. Being prepared ensures a smooth and stress-free experience on the big day.

5. Knowing the Hospital or Birthing Center: Familiarizing Yourself

If the birth will take place in a hospital or birthing center, familiarize yourself with the location and layout. This knowledge helps you navigate the facility efficiently during labor and delivery. Knowing the admission process and parking options can alleviate any last-minute concerns.

6. Being Attentive and Encouraging: Emotional Support

During labor, be attentive and encouraging, offering words of reassurance and comfort. Hold your partner's hand, provide a gentle massage, or simply be a steady presence by her side. Your emotional support during this challenging but miraculous event is invaluable.

7. *Advocating for Your Partner's Wishes: A Strong Advocate*

As the labor progresses, advocate for your partner's birthing preferences and choices. Communicate with the medical team, ensuring that her wishes are respected and followed to the best of the circumstances. Your advocacy reinforces her confidence and sense of control during labor.

<u>NOTE:</u>
Preparing for labor and delivery is a collaborative journey that strengthens your bond as a couple and prepares you both for the arrival of your baby. Attending childbirth education classes, creating a birth plan, and practicing breathing techniques empower you to actively participate and support your partner during labor.

Assembling a birthing bag and familiarizing yourself with the birthing location ensure a smooth and stress-free experience. Providing emotional support and advocating for your partner's wishes create a positive and nurturing environment for both her and your baby during this transformative and momentous event.

Embrace the journey of preparing for labor and delivery, knowing that your love and support make all the difference in creating a beautiful and meaningful birthing experience for your growing family. Your presence and encouragement as an expectant father are instrumental in helping your partner feel empowered, loved, and ready to welcome your child into the world.

CHAPTER 8

THE FIRST WEEKS WITH YOUR NEWBORN - Navigating the Whirlwind of New Parenthood

The first weeks with your newborn are an extraordinary time filled with wonder, love, and a whirlwind of emotions as you embark on the beautiful journey of parenthood. During this transformative period, you'll experience the magic of bonding with your baby and the challenges of adjusting to new routines and responsibilities. In these precious early days, understanding your baby's needs and prioritizing self-care are essential in creating a nurturing environment for both you and your newborn. Let us explore the key aspects of navigating the unique terrain of new parenthood and making the most of this special time.

Bonding with Your Baby: Creating a Connection that Lasts a Lifetime

The moment you cradle your newborn in your arms, an indescribable bond is formed. This magical connection is the foundation of building a secure and loving attachment with your baby. Through gentle touch, skin-to-skin contact, and nurturing gazes, you begin to develop a profound relationship with your little one, fostering a sense of security and trust that will shape their emotional well-being throughout life.

Navigating Sleep and Feeding Patterns: Embracing the New Rhythm

The first weeks with a newborn often involve adjusting to erratic sleep and feeding patterns. Understanding your baby's cues and needs is essential in establishing routines that work for both of you. By learning to recognize signs of hunger, tiredness, and comfort, you can provide the care and attention necessary to support your baby's growth and development while maintaining your own well-being.

Understanding Your Newborn's Cues: Communicating Without Words

Your baby communicates their needs through subtle cues and signals. Learning to interpret their nonverbal language is crucial in responding with sensitivity and care. From facial expressions to body movements, your newborn conveys a wealth of information that allows you to provide comfort and support when they need it most.

Taking Care of Yourself: Nurturing the New Parent

Amidst the joy and excitement of caring for your newborn, it's essential to prioritize self-care. As a new parent, taking time for yourself may seem challenging, but it is vital for your physical and emotional well-being. Seeking support from family and friends, finding moments of rest, and engaging in activities that bring you joy will recharge your energy and enable you to be the best version of yourself for your baby.

Creating a Calm and Soothing Environment: Supporting Your Baby's Development

A soothing environment is crucial for your baby's well-being. Creating a calm and comforting space for your newborn can have a profound impact on their sense of security and happiness. Soft lighting, gentle sounds, and skin-to-skin contact are all powerful ways to provide comfort and nurture your baby's emotional development.

The Power of Touch and Massage: Strengthening the Parent-Child Bond

Touch and massage are powerful ways to deepen the bond between parent and child. By incorporating gentle strokes and loving touch into your interactions with your baby, you not only promote relaxation and improve sleep but also strengthen the emotional connection between you and your little one.

Seeking Support and Connecting with Other Parents

During this transformative time, seeking support and connecting with other parents can be invaluable. Joining parenting groups, attending support classes, or simply talking to other new parents can provide reassurance and understanding as you navigate the joys and challenges of parenthood. Sharing experiences and advice with fellow parents can help you feel less alone and more supported on your journey.

Embracing Patience and Flexibility: Embracing the Learning Process

As a new parent, it's essential to embrace patience and flexibility. Parenthood is a journey of constant learning and adaptation. Embracing imperfections and being gentle with yourself will allow you to navigate the challenges of early parenthood with grace and understanding. Remember that every day is an opportunity to grow alongside your baby and to cherish the precious moments of their first weeks in this world.

<u>NOTE:</u>

The first weeks with your newborn are a time of profound transformation and unyielding love. By bonding with your baby, understanding their needs, and creating a soothing environment, you lay the groundwork for a strong and loving relationship. Navigating sleep and feeding patterns, prioritizing self-care, and seeking support from others will empower you to embrace the joys and challenges of early parenthood with confidence and grace.

By incorporating touch and massage into your interactions, you strengthen the bond between you and your baby, fostering a deep sense of connection. Embracing patience and flexibility as you adapt to the new role of parenthood will allow you to savor the unique journey of these first weeks with your newborn, cherishing the precious memories and forming an unbreakable bond that will endure for a lifetime.

CHAPTER 9

BALANCING WORK AND FAMILY LIFE - Nurturing Harmony in the Modern World

The delicate task of balancing work and family life is a universal challenge faced by many parents in today's fast-paced and interconnected world. The demands of professional responsibilities often intersect with the needs of family commitments, creating a delicate dance that requires careful navigation. Let us explore the complexities of finding harmony between your work and family roles. From managing time effectively to setting priorities and boundaries, we will explore practical strategies that empower you to create a balanced and fulfilling life for yourself and your loved ones.

Setting Priorities: Identifying What Truly Matters

In the quest for a work-life balance, setting clear priorities is essential. Take the time to reflect on what truly matters most to you and your family. While pursuing career goals is crucial, equally valuable are the cherished moments spent with your loved ones. By aligning your priorities, you can make conscious decisions that support your overall well-being and create a strong foundation for a harmonious work-life integration.

Time Management: Maximizing Productivity and Quality Time

Effective time management is the key to success in both your professional and family life. Utilize tools such as to-do lists, time blocks, and delegation to maximize productivity in your work. By efficiently managing your time, you create more space for quality moments with your family. Being fully present during these times allows you to nurture meaningful connections and build lasting memories.

Creating Boundaries: Learning to Say No

Learning to set boundaries is essential for maintaining a healthy work-life balance. While it can be tempting to take on additional commitments, saying no when necessary is a powerful act of self-care. By setting boundaries, you protect your family time and prioritize your well-being. Remember, it is okay to decline requests that may interfere with your ability to be present and supportive for your loved ones.

Flexible Work Arrangements: Finding Solutions for Work-Life Integration

In the pursuit of balance, consider exploring flexible work arrangements with your employer. Telecommuting, flextime, and other flexible options can offer valuable opportunities to achieve work-life integration. By advocating for family-friendly policies, you create a supportive work environment that acknowledges the importance of your family commitments alongside your professional responsibilities.

Prioritizing Self-Care: Nurturing Your Well-being

Amidst the juggling act of work and family life, do not forget to prioritize self-care. Taking care of yourself is not a luxury; it is a necessity. Carve out personal time to engage in activities that bring you joy, relaxation, and rejuvenation. By nurturing your well-being, you replenish your energy and become better equipped to care for your family and excel in your career.

Open Communication with Your Employer: Advocating for Family Support

Open communication with your employer is essential in creating a supportive work environment that recognizes the importance of family life. Discuss your family needs and advocate for family-friendly policies that benefit both you and your fellow colleagues. By fostering communication, you promote understanding and cooperation between your work and family spheres.

Embracing Imperfection: Being Kind to Yourself

It is important to embrace imperfection in the quest for work-life balance. Understand that achieving perfect balance is not always realistic, and that's okay. Be kind to yourself and let go of any unrealistic expectations. Embracing imperfection allows you to find peace in the ebb and flow of life's responsibilities, enabling you to navigate the complexities of work and family life with greater ease and self-compassion.

<u>**NOTE:**</u>

Balancing work and family life is an ongoing journey that requires self-awareness, prioritization, and intentional decision-making. By setting clear priorities, managing time effectively, and advocating for family support in the workplace, you create a foundation for a harmonious work-life integration. Prioritizing self-care and embracing imperfection empower you to navigate the challenges and joys of parenthood and career with resilience and grace.

Remember that the pursuit of work-life balance is not about achieving perfection but about nurturing a sense of harmony and fulfillment in both spheres of your life. By embracing the importance of work-life integration, you foster a nurturing environment for your well-being and the well-being of your loved ones. As you embark on this journey, know that with dedication and love, you can create a balanced and meaningful life that allows you to thrive both personally and professionally.

CHAPTER 10

BUILDING A STRONG PARENTING PARTNERSHIP AS AN EXPECTANT FATHER

As an expectant father, you are embarking on an incredible journey of parenthood alongside your partner. Building a strong parenting partnership is crucial in creating a nurturing and supportive environment for your child's growth and development. In this chapter, we will explore the key elements of fostering a strong parenting partnership with your partner, from effective communication and shared responsibilities to embracing teamwork and supporting each other's needs. By working together as a united front, you can navigate the joys and challenges of parenthood with confidence, love, and understanding.

1. *Effective Communication: The Foundation of a Strong Partnership*

Effective communication is the cornerstone of any successful parenting partnership. As expectant parents, open and honest dialogue allows you to express your hopes, fears, and expectations about parenthood. By actively listening to each other's thoughts and concerns, you can find common ground and create a unified approach to parenting that reflects both of your values and beliefs.

2. Shared Responsibilities: A Team Effort in Parenting

Parenting is a team effort that involves sharing responsibilities and working together to meet your child's needs. From prenatal care and preparing for the baby's arrival to diaper changes, feeding, and bedtime routines, collaborating as equal partners enhances your ability to provide a loving and stable environment for your child.

3. Embracing Each Other's Strengths: Recognizing Individual Contributions

Each parent brings unique strengths and qualities to the parenting partnership. Embrace and appreciate each other's strengths, whether it's your partner's nurturing nature or your own ability to calm the baby with ease. By recognizing and valuing each other's contributions, you create a harmonious and balanced parenting dynamic.

4. Teamwork in Decision Making: Parenting as a United Front

Decision making is an integral part of parenting. Discussing and making decisions together as a united front reinforces the sense of partnership in your parenting journey. Whether it's choosing a pediatrician, deciding on parenting strategies, or planning family outings, teamwork in decision making fosters a strong and cohesive parenting approach.

5. Supporting Each Other's Needs: Nurturing the Parent-Child Bond

As expectant parents, it's essential to support each other's emotional and physical needs. Take time to check in with one another, provide encouragement, and offer a helping hand when needed. By nurturing each other, you create a secure and loving environment that positively impacts the parent-child bond.

6. Flexibility and Adaptability: Navigating Parenthood's Ever-Changing Landscape

Parenthood is filled with surprises and unexpected challenges. Embrace flexibility and adaptability in your parenting partnership, as circumstances may change over time. Being open to adjusting your parenting approach allows you to grow together as parents and respond effectively to your child's evolving needs.

7. *Navigating Conflict with Respect and Empathy: Strengthening Your Connection*

Conflict is a natural part of any relationship, and parenthood may bring new challenges that require compromise and understanding. When conflicts arise, approach them with respect and empathy, seeking resolutions that benefit both you and your partner. By handling conflicts constructively, you reinforce the foundation of trust and love in your parenting partnership.

NOTE:

As an expectant father, building a strong parenting partnership with your partner is a rewarding and transformative experience. Effective communication, shared responsibilities, and embracing each other's strengths lay the groundwork for a unified and loving approach to parenting.

By working together as a team, supporting each other's needs, and navigating parenthood with flexibility and adaptability, you create a nurturing and stable environment for your child's well-being and development.

Handle conflicts with respect and empathy, fostering a deeper connection and understanding between you and your partner. Embrace the journey of building a strong parenting partnership with enthusiasm and love, knowing that by supporting and cherishing each other, you are creating a lasting bond that will enrich your child's life and your own in immeasurable ways. Parenthood is a beautiful adventure best experienced hand in hand, and as you embark on this journey together, the love and dedication you invest in your parenting partnership will shape the future of your growing family.

CHAPTER 11

GROWING AS A FATHER - Embracing the Ever-Changing Journey of Parenthood

Becoming a father marks the beginning of a transformative journey that continually evolves as your child grows. This chapter explores the joys, challenges, and opportunities for growth that come with embracing the role of a father. From nurturing the parent-child bond to evolving alongside your child's development, we delve into the key aspects of growing as a father and the profound impact you have on your child's life.

1. Nurturing the Parent-Child Bond: Cultivating Love and Trust

The parent-child bond is the foundation of your relationship with your child. Nurturing this bond involves cultivating love, trust, and emotional connection. Spending quality time together, engaging in meaningful conversations, and showing genuine interest in your child's life help strengthen this precious bond that will endure through the years.

2. Leading by Example: Becoming a Positive Role Model

As a father, you are a vital role model for your child. Your words and actions have a lasting impact on their character and values. Leading by example means demonstrating the qualities you wish to instill in your child, such as kindness, integrity, and resilience. By being a positive role model, you inspire your child to grow into the best version of themselves.

3. Embracing Communication: Building Trust and Understanding

Open and honest communication is the cornerstone of a strong parent-child relationship. Encouraging your child to share their thoughts and feelings without judgment fosters trust and understanding. Active listening and empathy create a safe space for your child to express themselves and feel heard, strengthening your bond and connection.

4. Encouraging Independence: Supporting Your Child's Growth

As your child grows, they will seek independence and explore the world around them. Encouraging their autonomy while providing a supportive environment empowers them to develop confidence and problem-solving skills. Be there to guide and offer assistance when needed, allowing your child to embrace new challenges with courage.

5. Cherishing Moments: Embracing the Magic of Fatherhood

Time passes swiftly, and childhood is fleeting. Cherish the moments with your child, from the ordinary to the extraordinary. Engage in their interests, celebrate their achievements, and be present in their lives. These cherished memories will create a profound and lasting connection between you and your child.

6. Learning and Growing Together: Evolving as a Father

Parenthood is a journey of continuous growth and learning for both you and your child. Embrace the opportunities for personal development and self-discovery that fatherhood presents. Be open to learning from your child, as they have unique perspectives and insights to share. Growing together strengthens the bond between father and child and enriches your relationship.

7. *Balancing Guidance and Support: Providing Unconditional Love*

Balancing guidance and support is essential in your role as a father. Set clear boundaries and expectations while offering unconditional love and understanding. Provide a safe and nurturing environment for your child to learn and make mistakes, knowing that you are there to support them no matter what.

Note:

Growing as a father is an ever-changing and beautiful journey filled with love, growth, and shared experiences. Nurturing the parent-child bond, leading by example, and embracing open communication create a strong and loving foundation for your relationship with your child.

As your child grows and explores the world, encourage their independence while cherishing the precious moments spent together. Embrace the magic of fatherhood and the continuous learning and growth it brings.

Balancing guidance and support, you provide your child with the tools to navigate life while knowing they have your unwavering love and backing. Embrace the evolving journey of parenthood with enthusiasm and dedication, knowing that you play a profound and irreplaceable role in shaping your child's life and future.

CHAPTER 12

MAKING MEMORIES AND HAVING FUN - Creating Lasting Bonds with Your Child

As a father, one of the most rewarding aspects of parenthood is the opportunity to make memories and have fun with your child. This chapter explores the significance of creating lasting bonds through shared experiences, joyful moments, and meaningful adventures. From playtime and family outings to special traditions and spontaneous laughter, we delve into the essence of making memories and cherishing the time spent with your child. These cherished moments not only strengthen your relationship but also become the building blocks of a loving and connected family.

1. Embracing Playtime: Building Connections through Fun

Playtime is a magical space where you and your child can bond, laugh, and explore the wonders of the world together. Engaging in imaginative play, building with blocks, or playing games cultivates a sense of connection and fosters your child's emotional development. Embrace your inner child and be fully present during these moments, savoring the joy of play with your little one.

2. Family Outings and Adventures: Creating Shared Experiences

Family outings and adventures offer the perfect opportunity to create shared experiences and lasting memories. Whether it's exploring nature, visiting a museum, or going on a picnic, these outings strengthen your family bond and provide a sense of togetherness. The memories created during these special moments become cherished stories that you and your child will treasure for a lifetime.

3. Special Traditions: Building a Sense of Belonging

Establishing special traditions fosters a sense of belonging and reinforces your family's unique identity. Whether it's a weekly family movie night, holiday traditions, or yearly vacations, these rituals create a strong sense of connection and anticipation. Traditions provide stability and comfort while allowing you to celebrate the joys of being a family.

4. Spontaneous Laughter and Silly Moments: Finding Joy in the Everyday

Life is full of unexpected moments of laughter and silliness, and embracing these moments with your child deepens your bond. From silly dances and tickle fights to funny faces and inside jokes, these spontaneous moments of joy create a sense of lightheartedness and love in your family dynamic.

5. Capturing Moments: Preserving Memories for Generations

In the digital age, capturing moments has become easier than ever. Take the time to document special occasions, milestones, and everyday adventures through photographs and videos. These visual memories serve as a tangible reminder of the love and happiness shared within your family and can be cherished for generations to come.

6. Quality Time: Being Present and Engaged

Amidst the busyness of life, prioritize quality time with your child. Being fully present and engaged during your interactions creates a sense of value and importance for your child. Put away distractions and give your undivided attention, showing them that they are cherished and loved.

7. Embracing New Experiences: Expanding Horizons Together

Explore new experiences with your child, introducing them to different activities, cultures, and hobbies. Embracing new experiences together not only broadens your child's horizons but also strengthens your bond as you share the excitement and curiosity of discovery.

Note

Making memories and having fun with your child is an integral part of being a father. Embracing playtime, sharing family outings and adventures, and establishing special traditions create a sense of love and togetherness within your family.

Spontaneous laughter and capturing moments preserve the joy and happiness of shared experiences for years to come. Prioritize quality time, being present and engaged in your interactions, to create a deep sense of connection and value for your child.

Embrace new experiences together, expanding horizons and fostering a sense of curiosity and wonder. The memories created during these moments become the fabric of your family's story, creating lasting bonds that enrich your lives and create a loving and connected family unit. As you make memories and have fun with your child, know that you are building a treasure trove of moments that will be cherished and celebrated for a lifetime.

CHAPTER 13

PARENTING THROUGH CHALLENGES - Navigating the Storms with Resilience

Parenthood is a journey filled with ups and downs, and as a father, you will inevitably face various challenges along the way. This chapter explores the art of parenting through challenging times, acknowledging that difficulties are a natural part of the parenting experience. From coping with stress and overcoming obstacles to fostering resilience and seeking support, we delve into the key aspects of navigating these storms with strength and love. Embracing challenges as opportunities for growth enables you to become a steadfast and compassionate father for your child.

1. Coping with Stress: Prioritizing Self-Care

Parenting can be demanding and stressful, and it's essential to prioritize self-care during challenging times. Take time for yourself to recharge and replenish your energy. Engage in activities that bring you joy and relaxation, allowing you to approach challenges with a clear and focused mind.

2. Overcoming Obstacles: Embracing Problem-Solving

Obstacles are an inevitable part of parenting. Embrace problem-solving as a tool to address challenges effectively. Approach challenges with a positive mindset, focusing on solutions rather than dwelling on the problems. By demonstrating resilience and determination, you set a powerful example for your child to follow.

3. Fostering Resilience: Bouncing Back with Strength

Resilience is the ability to bounce back from adversity with strength and grace. As a father, fostering resilience in yourself and your child is essential. Model resilience by acknowledging setbacks and demonstrating how to overcome them. Encourage your child to face challenges and support them as they navigate difficult situations.

4. Seeking Support: The Power of Connection

Seeking support from loved ones, friends, or professionals can be transformative during challenging times. Reach out for help when needed, as sharing your struggles can provide valuable insights and reassurance. Remember that you don't have to face challenges alone, and seeking support is a sign of strength, not weakness.

5. Maintaining Open Communication: A Safe Space for Expression

During challenging times, maintain open communication with your child. Create a safe space for them to express their feelings and concerns without judgment. Be attentive and empathetic, reassuring your child that their emotions are valid and understood.

6. Embracing Flexibility: Adapting to Changing Circumstances

Flexibility is key when navigating challenges in parenthood. Embrace the need for adaptation and be open to change. Be willing to adjust your approach as circumstances evolve, understanding that flexibility allows you to meet the needs of your child and family in the best possible way.

7. Practicing Patience and Compassion: A Nurturing Presence

Practicing patience and compassion during challenging times is a gift you can give yourself and your child. Be gentle with yourself as you navigate the difficulties of parenthood. Show understanding and compassion toward your child as they navigate their own emotions and challenges.

Parenting through challenges is an integral part of being a father. Coping with stress, overcoming obstacles, and fostering resilience empower you to navigate difficult times with strength and determination. Seeking support and maintaining open communication create a network of understanding and compassion that sustains you through the storm.

Embracing flexibility and practicing patience enable you to adapt to changing circumstances and provide a nurturing presence for your child. Remember that facing challenges is an opportunity for growth and learning, both for you and your child.

As you navigate the storms of parenthood with resilience and love, know that your dedication and unwavering support create a stable and loving environment for your child to flourish. Embrace challenges as a catalyst for growth, and your journey as a father will be filled with the depth and richness of experience that shapes your child's life in profound ways.

CHAPTER 14

EMBRACING FATHERHOOD - The Journey of Love and Transformation

Fatherhood is a transformative journey that touches the depths of the heart and soul. This chapter explores the essence of embracing fatherhood with love, dedication, and a sense of purpose. From the joys of bonding with your child to the responsibilities of nurturing their growth, we delve into the profound impact of fatherhood on your life and the lives of those you hold dear. Embrace the role of a father with an open heart, knowing that this journey will shape you in ways you never imagined.

1. Bonding with Your Child: The Power of Connection

The bond between a father and child is a treasure beyond measure. Embrace the joys of bonding with your child through shared experiences, heartfelt conversations, and moments of play. Your presence and love create a secure foundation that nourishes your child's emotional well-being.

2. Embracing Vulnerability: The Strength in Openness

As a father, embracing vulnerability is a testament to your strength. Openly expressing your emotions and being receptive to your child's feelings create an environment of trust and understanding. Embrace vulnerability as a gateway to deepening your connection with your child and those around you.

3. Learning and Growing Together: A Journey of Mutual Discovery

Fatherhood is a journey of learning and growing, not just for your child but also for you. Embrace the lessons your child teaches you and the wisdom they bring into your life. Embrace the opportunity to grow alongside your child as you both navigate the adventure of life.

4. Celebrating Uniqueness: Embracing Your Child's Individuality

Each child is unique, with their own interests, talents, and dreams. Embrace and celebrate your child's individuality, supporting their passions and aspirations. Your acceptance and encouragement empower them to embrace their true selves with confidence.

5. Nurturing Love and Support: A Safe Haven for Your Child

As a father, your love and support create a safe haven for your child to thrive. Offer encouragement during challenges, celebrate their achievements, and be a constant source of reassurance. Your unwavering love provides a solid foundation from which they can explore the world with courage.

6. Leading with Empathy: Understanding Your Child's Perspective

Empathy is a guiding light in fatherhood. Seek to understand your child's perspective, acknowledging their emotions and experiences with compassion. Leading with empathy fosters open communication and strengthens the bond between you and your child.

7. Cherishing Moments: The Gift of Presence

The moments shared with your child are precious and fleeting. Embrace the gift of presence by being fully engaged in their lives. Cherish the small moments of joy, laughter, and growth, knowing that these memories will forever hold a special place in your heart.

Note:

Embracing fatherhood is a journey of love, growth, and transformation. The bond you forge with your child is a profound connection that shapes both of your lives. Embrace vulnerability as a strength and celebrate your child's uniqueness with unconditional love and support.

Learn and grow alongside your child, cherishing the moments that make your journey as a father truly meaningful. Leading with empathy and understanding creates a nurturing environment that enables your child to flourish and become the best version of themselves.

As you embrace fatherhood with an open heart and a sense of purpose, know that the love and dedication you invest in your child's life will leave a lasting legacy that transcends time. Embrace this beautiful journey of fatherhood, for it is a gift that enriches your life in ways beyond imagination.

CHAPTER 15

ADVICE FROM EXPERIENCED DADS - Pearls of Wisdom from the Journey of Fatherhood

In this chapter, we seek wisdom from seasoned fathers who have navigated the beautiful journey of parenthood. Their insights and advice are invaluable gems that offer guidance and reassurance to expectant fathers. From handling the challenges of fatherhood to cherishing the joys and lessons learned, the experiences shared by these fathers provide a wealth of knowledge for those about to embark on this transformative path.

Advice from Experienced Dads:

1. *Embrace the Unpredictability:* Fatherhood is filled with surprises and unexpected moments. Embrace the unpredictability and be flexible in your approach as a father. Allow yourself to be present and relish every moment, even amidst the chaos.

2. *Prioritize Quality Time:* In the midst of busy schedules, prioritize quality time with your child. Create special rituals or routines that strengthen your bond and create lasting memories.

3. *Be Patient with Yourself:* Fatherhood is a learning curve. Be patient with yourself as you adapt to your new role. Embrace the journey of growth, and know that mistakes are a natural part of the process.

4. *Listen to Your Child*: Truly listen to your child, for their thoughts and feelings are valuable. Show genuine interest in their world, and be present in the moments when they need your support and understanding.

5. *Seek Support:* Reach out to other fathers or support networks. Parenting can be challenging, but knowing you are not alone in your experiences can make a world of difference.

6. *Embrace Playfulness:* Don't forget to have fun and be playful with your child. Letting your inner child shine through strengthens your connection and creates a loving environment.

Short Stories of Experiences:

1. The First Steps:

David, an expectant father, recalled a heartwarming moment when his daughter took her first steps. He had been anxiously awaiting this milestone and couldn't contain his excitement when he witnessed her wobbly yet determined strides. Tears filled his eyes as he scooped her up in his arms, realizing that he was witnessing one of many milestones that would shape their bond as father and daughter.

2. The Bedtime Ritual:

Michael, a seasoned father of two, shared his bedtime ritual with his children. Each night, he would gather his kids in their cozy pajamas and read them bedtime stories. He cherished these quiet moments of togetherness, where they would embark on adventures through the pages of their favorite books. This ritual not only instilled a love for reading in his children but also created a special time for them to unwind and feel safe in their father's embrace.

3. Finding Strength in Challenges:

John, a father of three, recalled the challenges he faced when juggling a demanding job and family life. During a particularly trying time, his youngest child fell ill, and he had to take time off work to care for them. Despite the stress and uncertainties, John found strength in being present for his child's recovery. He realized that in those challenging moments, his role as a father was his most significant responsibility, and everything else could wait.

4. The Joy of Shared Hobbies:

Tom, an avid outdoorsman, shared his love for fishing with his teenage son, Mark. They spent weekends by the lake, fishing and sharing stories. Through their shared hobby, Tom and Mark formed a deep connection and mutual respect for each other's interests. The quiet moments by the water not only brought them closer but also provided a space for open conversations about life's challenges and triumphs.

Note

The advice and experiences of experienced dads offer invaluable insights for expectant fathers embarking on the journey of fatherhood. Embrace the unpredictability and cherish every moment with your child. Prioritize quality time and listen to your child's thoughts and feelings. Seek support when needed and don't forget to be playful and have fun. The short stories of fathers' experiences remind us of the beauty and significance of this transformative journey of fatherhood. Embrace the joys, the challenges, and the moments of growth with an open heart, knowing that you are building a loving and lasting connection with your child that will enrich both of your lives in immeasurable ways.